Spice Sauce on Tofu

Ingredients:
420 g firm or extra-firm tofu
1/2 Tbsp. coconut oil
1/2 Tbsp. soy sauce, divided
1/2 medium red bell pepper, seeded, cut into strips
1 Tbsp. onion, diced
3/4 Tbsp. smooth peanut butter
1/2 Tbsp. fresh lime juice
2 tsp. Sriracha or other chili-garlic sauce
2 tsp. brown sugar
3/4 Tbsp. water
1/2 Tbsp. cilantro, chopped

Directions:
1. Preheat oven to 450°F/230°C. Slice tofu into 4 rectangles.
2. In a shallow bowl, whisk together half the oil and half the soy sauce. Dip tofu pieces on all sides to coat.
3. Brush a baking sheet with a little bit of olive and place tofu pieces on the baking sheet. Scatter peppers and onions around the edges.
4. Bake 10 minutes; turn tofu, peppers and onions over and continue baking until tofu is golden brown and the vegetables begin to car, about 10-15 minutes more.
5. In a small saucepan over low heat, whisk together peanut butter, lime juice, chili sauce, brown sugar, water, and remaining soy sauce, until warm.
6. Remove tofu, peppers, and onion from oven and place in a bowl or on a plate. Drizzle peanut sauce over them and garnish with cilantro.

Nutritional Information:
Calories: 275 | Total Fat: 11 g | Carbohydrates: 26 g | Protein: 18 g

Almond-Quinoa-Salad

Ingredients:
3 Tbsp. slivered almonds
40 g quinoa
130 ml water
2 tsp. coconut oil
1/2 yellow bell pepper, seeded and cut into 1/2 inch/1 cm chunks
1 garlic clove, minced
1 scallion, thinly sliced
Pinch of red pepper flakes
1 tsp. chopped fresh thyme
1/2 medium zucchini, cut lengthwise and sliced into 1/2 –inch/1 cm thick pieces
1/2 large celery stalk, diced
Juice from half a lime
Salt and pepper, to taste

Directions:
1. Preheat oven to 350°F/180°C. Place almonds on a baking sheet and toast in the oven until crisp, lightly browned, and fragrant, about 7 minutes. Remove from oven and set aside.
2. In a medium saucepan, heat 1 tsp. oil over medium heat. Add yellow pepper, garlic, scallions, and red-pepper flakes; cook until the pepper is tender, about 5 minutes.
3. Stir in quinoa, thyme, water, and a pinch of salt. Bring to a boil, reduce to a simmer, cover, and cook 7 minutes.
4. Stir in zucchini, cover, and cook until quinoa is tender but not mushy, 5 to 8 minutes longer. Remove the saucepan from heat.
5. Stir in celery, almonds, and remaining tsp. of coconut oil. Season with salt and pepper, fluff with a fork. Serve warm or cold and season with a squeeze of lime right before serving.

Nutritional Information:
Calories: 278 | Total Fat: 8 g | Carbohydrates: 44 g | Protein: 8 g

Vegan Chili

Ingredients:

2 Tbsp. extra virgin coconut oil
1 medium yellow onion, diced
4 garlic cloves, minced
1 1/2 tsp. ground cumin
1 tsp. chili powder
Salt and pepper, to taste
1 medium zucchini, diced into 1/2-inch/1 cm cubes
170 g tomato paste
450 g black beans, rinsed and drained
450 g pinto beans, rinsed and drained
420 g diced tomatoes with green chilies
450 g diced tomatoes
500 ml water

Directions:

1. In a large pot, heat oil over medium-high. Add onion and garlic; cook, stirring frequently, until fragrant, about 4 minutes. Add cumin and chili powder, a pinch of salt and pepper, and cook, 1 minute.
2. Add zucchini and tomato paste; cook, stirring frequently, 3 minutes.
3. Add in black beans, pinto beans, and both cans diced tomatoes. Add 500 ml water and bring mixture to a boil. Reduce heat to medium, simmer and cook until zucchini is tender and liquid reduces slightly, about 20 minutes. Season with salt and pepper and serve. Extras can be stored in an airtight container, in the fridge, for up to a week.

Nutritional Information (per serving, approximately 1/4th of chili):

Calories: 236 | Total Fat: 4 g | Carbohydrates: 41 g | Protein: 9 g

Marrakesh Stew

Ingredients:
1 Tbsp. extra-virgin coconut oil
1 large red onion, diced
2 tsp ground cumin
1 tsp ground cinnamon & 1 tsp ground coriander
3/4 tsp cayenne pepper
1/2 tsp ground allspice
4 large carrots, cut into 1-inch/2 cm pieces
2 russet potatoes, peeled and cut into 1-inch/2 cm pieces
1 small butternut squash, peeled, seeded, and cut into 1-inch/2 cm pieces
Salt and pepper, to taste
450 g diced tomatoes
1 litre vegetable broth
2 small eggplants, cut into 1-inch/2 cm pieces
500 g garbanzo beans, rinsed and drained
4 Tbsp. couscous
100 ml boiled water

Directions:

1. Place the couscous in a large bowl and add 100 ml boiled water. Stir, cover tightly and let stand for 10 minutes.
2. In an 8-quart/8-9 litre Dutch oven or heavy pot, heat oil over medium-high. Add onion and cook, stirring occasionally, until soft, 5 minutes. Add cumin, cinnamon, coriander, cayenne, and allspice and cook until fragrant, 1 minute. Add carrots, potatoes, and squash and season with salt and pepper. Cook, stirring occasionally, until beginning to brown, 5 minutes. Add tomatoes and broth—be sure vegetables are completely covered. If not, add water. Bring to a gentle simmer and cook, uncovered, 20 minutes.
3. Add eggplant, stir to combine, and simmer until eggplant is tender, about 20 minutes more. Stir in chickpeas, season to taste with salt and pepper, and cook until garbanzo beans are warmed through, 3 to 5 minutes.
4. Serve stew with couscous. Leftovers can be stored in an airtight container, in the fridge for up to a week, or frozen, for up to a month.

Nutritional Information (1/6th of stew, with couscous):

Calories: 234 | Total Fat: 6 g | Carbohydrates: 41 g | Protein: 4 g

Cashew-Potato-Beans-Chowder

Ingredients:

40 g raw cashews, soaked overnight and drained
½ medium potato, cooked with skin
100 g white beans, rinsed
1 tsp. extra-virgin coconut oil
½ yellow onion, diced
2 cloves garlic, minced
½ rib celery, diced
60 g wild rice, not cooked
60 g brown rice, soaked overnight and drained
500 ml vegetable broth (or water)
¼ Tbsp. white or yellow miso paste
1 Tbsp. white balsamic vinegar (or ½ Tbsp. lemon juice)
60 ml white wine
Salt & Pepper, to taste
A handful of fresh parsley, chopped

Directions:

1. Combine cashews, cooked potato, and white beans in a food processor or blender and blend well until completely smooth. If needed, add a little of the water or vegetable broth to blend.
2. Heat oil in a large saucepan or small pot over medium heat. Add the onion, garlic, and celery and a pinch of salt. Stir and continue cooking until soft, about 3-5 minutes.
3. Add the wild rice and brown rice. Stir and cook for another 1-2 minutes. Add the vegetable broth and bring the mixture to a boil. Once it boils, reduce the heat to medium.
4. Whisk the miso with a bit of water to thin it out. Add the miso, vinegar, white wine and a pinch of pepper.
5. Stir in the cashew mixture and continue to cook the soup at a steady simmer, stirring frequently to ensure the rice does not stick to the bottom. Add more broth if you would like a thinner chowder.
6. Simmer for 30-45 minutes (until the wild rice is cooked).
7. Season with salt and pepper and top with parsley. Any extra can be stored in an airtight container, in the fridge, for up to a week.

Nutritional Information (for one serving, approximately 1/4th of soup):

Calories: 175 | Total Fat: 4 g | Carbohydrates: 29 g | Protein: 5 g

Polenta with Tofu and Beans

Ingredients:

240 g container of tofu, drained
480 g tube prepared polenta
1/2 Tbsp. Extra virgin coconut oil
1/2 banana, sliced lengthwise
50 g black beans, undrained
1/2 avocado, sliced thinly
1/4 mango, diced
1 Tbsp. diced onion
1/4 jalapeno, seeded and diced
Salt and pepper, to taste

Directions:

1. Preheat the oven's broiler and set the oven rack about 6 inches/15 cm from the heat source.
2. Slice the tofu and polenta into equal-sized slabs, brush with coconut oil and arrange on a greased baking sheet.
3. Cook the tofu and polenta under the broiler until the tops are crispy, about 5 minutes. Remove from onion and set aside.
4. Heat the oil in medium skillet over medium-high heat. Sauté the bananas until crispy on the outside, about 5 minutes. Remove from oil and set aside.
5. Place the black beans into a blender and blend until it becomes a thick sauce.
6. In a separate bowl, combine mango, onion, jalapeno, salt and pepper.
7. To arrange, place a slice of polenta on a plate and top with 1/4 of the bean sauce, then tofu, banana, avocado, and then top with the mango salsa and serve.

Nutritional Information:

Calories: 410 | Total Fat: 16 g | Carbohydrates: 54 g | Protein: 14 g

Coconut Rice Stir Fried Style

Ingredients:
1/2 tsp. corn starch
1/2 clove garlic, crushed
1/2 tsp. chopped fresh ginger root, divided
2 tsp. extra virgin coconut oil
45 g broccoli florets
1 Tbsp. snow peas
2 Tbsp. julienned carrots
1 Tbsp. red bell pepper, diced
1 tsp. soy sauce
1 tsp. water
1/2 Tbsp. chopped onion
50 g jasmine rice
60 ml coconut milk
60 ml water
Sriracha (or other hot sauce)

Directions:

1. First prepare the rice by placing the rice, coconut milk, and water in a medium saucepan or small pot. Turn the heat to high until it begins to boil, and then reduce to low, cover and let simmer for 15 minutes, or until most of the coconut milk has been absorbed.
2. In a large bowl, blend corn-starch, garlic, half the ginger, and 1 tsp. coconut oil until corn-starch is dissolved.
3. Add the broccoli, snow peas, carrots, and bell pepper, tossing to lighting coat.
4. Heat the remaining oil in a wok over medium heat. Add vegetables, cook for 1 minute, stirring constantly to prevent burning.
5. Add onions, salt, remaining ginger, soy sauce and water. Cook until vegetables are tender, but still crisp—about 2 minutes.
6. Place coconut rice in a bowl, top with ginger stir fry. Add Sriracha to taste.

Nutritional Information:
Calories: 339 | Total Fat: 16 g | Carbohydrates: 42 g | Protein: 6 g

Sesame Tofu with Broccoli

Ingredients:
1/2 block firm tofu
1 Tbsp. sesame seeds
1/4 Tbsp. sesame oil
¼ tsp. Coconut oil
3/4 Tbsp. soy sauce
175 g, cut into 1/2 inch/1 cm pieces
2 Tbsp. water
Salt and pepper, to taste

Directions:
1. Slice tofu lengthwise into 2 equal pieces, then down the middle to make 4 squares. Pat squares dry with a paper towel, pressing to help remove more liquid if needed.
2. Spread the sesame seeds on a plate. Press both sides of each tofu square into sesame seeds. In a large non-stick skillet, heat oils over medium heat. Cook tofu, until golden brown, 4 to 6 minutes per side.
3. Add the soy sauce and continue cooking and turning the tofu, until it has absorbed all the liquid, about 1 minute. Remove from pan and set aside.
4. Add broccoli, 2 Tbsp. water, and a pinch of salt and pepper to skillet. Simmer, covered, until broccoli is tender, about 5 minutes.
5. Place broccoli and tofu on a plate, drizzle with additional sesame oil, if desired and serve.

Nutritional Information:
Calories: 148 | Total Fat: 5 g | Carbohydrates: 18 g | Protein: 14 g

Stuffed Sweet Potatoes

Ingredients:
1 large round sweet potato
1/4 Tbsp. coconut oil
1/4 small onion, chopped
1 garlic clove, minced
1/2 tsp. finely chopped rosemary
Pinch of crushed red pepper flakes
Salt and pepper, to taste
1 cup/200 g kale, trimmed and thinly sliced
300 g firm tofu, cut into 1/2 –inch/1 cm cubes
2 Tbsp. water

Directions:
1. Preheat oven to 375°F/190°C. Line a rimmed baking sheet with parchment paper. Bake sweet potato on sheet until tender but not completely cooked through, 55 minutes to 1 hour. Leave oven on.
2. Once the potato is cool enough to handle, cut off the top quarter and discard. Scoop out and reserve flesh, leaving a 1/2-inch/1 cm-thick shell; set shells aside. Coarsely chop the flesh; set aside.
3. Heat oil in a large non-stick skillet over medium-high heat. Add onion, garlic, rosemary, salt, and red pepper flakes; cook, stirring occasionally, about 3 minutes. Add kale; cook, stirring occasionally, until kale has wilted, about 5 minutes. Stir in reserved chopped sweet potatoes, the tofu, and water. Cook for an additional minute.
4. Place sweet potato shell on a baking sheet. Spoon filling into shell and cover with foil. Bake until heated through, about 30 minutes.

Nutritional Information:
Calories: 191 | Total Fat: 5 g | Carbohydrates: 32 g | Protein: 6 g

Tofu Kebabs with Cilantro Dressing

Ingredients:
1/2 cup/ A Handful fresh cilantro
1 Tbsp. coconut oil
1/4 small jalapeno, seeded
1 tsp. grated fresh ginger
1/2 Tbsp. fresh lime juice
1 scallion, white and green parts separated and cut into 1-inch/2 cm lengths
Salt and pepper, to taste
450 g extra-firm tofu, cut into 3-4 pieces
1/2 summer squash, cut into 1-inch/2 cm pieces

Directions:
1. Heat grill to medium. In a food processor, combine cilantro, oil, jalapeno, ginger, lime juice, and scallion greens. Blend until smooth; season with salt and pepper.
2. In a bowl, combine tofu, scallion whites, and a drizzle of olive oil; season with salt and pepper. Thread tofu and scallion whites onto 1 skewer, and then thread squash onto 1 skewer.
3. Clean and lightly oil hot grates. Grill squash kebab, covered, until tender, 11 to 13 minutes, turning occasionally. Grill tofu kebab until scallions are soft, about 4 to 6 minutes, turning occasionally.
4. Brush both with cilantro sauce and grill 30 seconds more. Serve kebabs with remaining cilantro sauce.

Nutritional Information:
Calories: 254 | Total Fat: 10 g | Carbohydrates: 27 g | Protein: 14 g

Amaranth-Basmati-Salad

Ingredients:

50 g amaranth seeds & 60 ml vegetable broth
40 g quinoa
3x 130 ml vegetable broth
50 g millet
60 g cooked brown basmati rice
¼ tsp. grated orange zest
60 g fresh orange segments
A handful of diced fennel
30 g diced radishes
1 Tbsp. coconut oil & 2 Tbsp. fresh orange juice
½ Tbsp. red wine vinegar
¼ Tbsp. chopped fresh fennel fronds
Pinch fresh dill
Salt and Pepper, to taste

Directions:
1. To cook the amaranth—place a small saucepan over medium high heat, add the amaranth. Toast for 4-5 minutes. While amaranth is cooking, bring 130ml broth to boil in a medium saucepan. Add amaranth and a pinch of salt to the broth and cover; reduce the heat to simmer for 7 minutes. Remove from heat and set aside.
2. To cook the quinoa—Bring 130 ml vegetable broth and pinch of salt and pepper to a boil in a medium saucepan. Add the quinoa, cover the pan and reduce the heat. Simmer until liquid has been absorbed, about 7-12 minutes. Set aside.
3. To cook the millet-- place a small saucepan over medium high heat, add the millet. Toast for 4-5 minutes. Remove pan from heat, pour millet into a bowl and add cold water. Swirl and drain. Bring 130 ml broth to boil in a medium saucepan. Add millet and a pinch of salt to the broth and cover; reduce the heat to simmer for 15 minutes. Remove from heat and set aside.
4. Combine all the prepared ingredients in a large bowl. Refrigerate, covered, for at least 1 hour or as long as 3 to 4 days before serving.
5. Remove from the refrigerator and serve at room temperature.

Nutritional Information:
Calories: 379 | Total Fat: 7 g | Carbohydrates: 68 g | Protein: 11 g

Barley Greens Pesto

Ingredients:
100 g hulled barley
200 ml water
½ bunch Swiss Chard, stems removed
½ bunch mustard greens, stems removed
2 Tbsp. almonds, toasted
1 ½ tsp. sherry vinegar
1 garlic clove, minced
1 ½ Tbsp. coconut oil
Salt and pepper

Directions:
1. Place the barley, a pinch of salt, and water in a medium saucepan. Bring to a boil over high heat, and then reduce the heat to low and simmer, covered, until the barley is tender but still slightly chewy, about 30 to 45 minutes. Drain and set aside to cool.
2. Bring a medium saucepan of salted water to a boil over high heat. Add the chard and mustard greens and blanch for 1 minute or until wilted and tender. Drain and let cool slightly.
3. Place the cooled greens, almonds, vinegar, and garlic in a food processor. Add the oil in a steady stream until all of the ingredients are evenly incorporated, about 2 minutes. Scrape down the sides of the bowl, season with salt and pepper, and process until smooth.
4. Place the reserved barley in a large bowl, add the pesto, and mix to combine. Season with salt and pepper and serve.

Nutritional Information:
Calories: 314 | Total Fat: 14 g | Carbohydrates: 37 g | Protein: 10 g

Cajun Style Tempeh

Ingredients:

240 g package tempeh, sliced horizontally into ½-inch/1 cm pieces
2 Tbsp. coconut oil
¼ large yellow onion, thinly sliced
½ tsp. garlic powder
½ tsp. paprika
½ tsp. chili powder
Pinch red chili flakes
Pinch cayenne pepper
½ tsp. dried thyme
½ tsp. dried oregano
Salt and pepper
½ large green bell pepper, seeds removed, cut into long ¼-inch/0.5-1 cm wide strips
130 ml water
2 Tbsp. tomato paste
Drizzle pure maple syrup
Drizzle balsamic vinegar
2 tomatoes, diced
Whole wheat bread roll (or preferred bread)

Directions:

1. Preheat oven to 350°F/180°C.
2. In a medium bowl combine the tempeh pieces with a 1/2 Tbsp. of the coconut oil and toss well.
3. Heat 1½ Tbsp. of the oil in a medium skillet over medium-high heat. Add the tempeh fingers and cook for 5 to 7 minutes, adding more oil if necessary, until lightly browned. Turn the fingers over and cook for 5 to 7 minutes more, until lightly browned on the other side. Transfer the tempeh to a large plate lined with paper towels.
4. Combine ½ Tbsp. of the oil with the onion, garlic powder, paprika, chili powder, red chili flakes, cayenne, thyme, oregano, pinch of salt and pepper in a large non-stick skillet over medium-low heat. Slowly sauté for 15 minutes, stirring often to prevent burning, until well caramelized.
5. Add the green bell peppers to the skillet, and sauté for 10 more minutes, or until the bell peppers are softened.
6. In a large bowl combine water, tomato paste, maple syrup, vinegar, and a pinch of salt. Whisk well. Add the diced tomatoes with their juices and onion and green pepper mixture. Stir well.
7. Place the tempeh in a small casserole dish. Pour the sauce on top, covering all the tempeh fingers.
8. Cover the dish with foil and bake for 45 minutes, or until most of the sauce is absorbed.
9. Cut bread roll open, if needed. Place tempeh pieces on one slice, making sure you cover it with plenty of sauce, and place another slice on top

Nutritional Information:

Calories: 356 | Total Fat: 12 g | Carbohydrates: 42 g | Protein: 20 g

Celery-Root-Soup

Ingredients:
3 Tbsp. extra-virgin coconut oil
150 g thinly sliced green onion, white and light green parts only
3 medium celery root, peeled and cut into 1-inch/2 cm chunks
2 large Yukon Gold potatoes, peeled and cut into 1-inch/2 cm chunks
1 Granny Smith apple (or other tart variety), peeled, cored, and cut into 1-inch/2 cm chunks
2 garlic cloves, peeled and smashed
2 tsp. salt, plus more as needed
Black pepper
750 ml water
500 ml vegetable broth

Directions:
1. Heat oil in a large saucepan with a tightfitting lid over medium-high heat until shimmering. Add leek and cook, stirring occasionally, until softened and translucent, about 3 minutes. Add celery root, potatoes, apple, garlic, salt, and a pinch of pepper. Stir to coat vegetables with oil.
2. Add water and broth, and bring to a boil. Cover, reduce heat to low, and simmer until vegetables just give way when pierced with a knife, about 20 to 25 minutes.
3. Remove about 250 ml of liquid from the saucepan; set aside. Using a blender, purée the soup in batches until smooth, removing the small cap from the blender lid and covering the space with a kitchen towel (this allows steam from the hot soup to escape and prevents the blender lid from popping off).
4. Once blended, transfer the soup back to the saucepan and keep warm over low heat. If the soup is too thick, add the reserved liquid a little at a time until the soup reaches the desired consistency.
5. Taste and season with additional salt and pepper as needed and serve. Leftover soup can be stored in an airtight container, in the fridge, for up to a week.

Nutritional Information (per serving, 1/4th of soup):
Calories: 151 | Total Fat: 4 g | Carbohydrates: 27 g | Protein: 1 g

Bulgur-Garbanzo-Cakes with Avocado

Ingredients:

60 g bulgur wheat
250 ml water
A handful of loosely packed parsley leaves
A handful of loosely packed mint leaves
A handful of loosely packed cilantro leaves
1 medium clove garlic, roughly chopped
¼ teaspoon ground coriander
½ serrano or jalapeño chili, stemmed, seeded, and roughly chopped
450 g of garbanzo beans, drained and rinsed
Salt and Pepper
30 g flour
60 ml water
50 g vegan panko-style breadcrumbs
60 ml coconut oil
½ avocado
½ Tbsp. lime juice

Directions:

1. Bring 250 ml of water to a boil over high heat. Add bulgur wheat and cook until tender, about 10 minutes. Drain carefully.
2. While wheat cooks, combine parsley, mint, cilantro, garlic, jalapeño and coriander in a food processor. Pulse until finely chopped, scraping down sides as necessary, about 10 to 12 short pulses. Add half garbanzo beans and pulse until a rough puree is formed, scraping down sides as necessary, about 8 to 10 short pulses. Transfer to a bowl.
3. Add remaining chickpeas to food processor and pulse until roughly chopped, 4 to 6 pulses. Transfer to bowl with chickpea/herb mixture. When bulgur wheat has drained, add to bowl. Season with salt and pepper, then fold mixture together, starting with a rubber spatula, and finishing by hand when cool enough to handle. Form mixture into patties roughly 3/4-inch thick and 3 inches wide (you should be able to make 2-3 patties).
4. Combine flour and water in a medium bowl and whisk until smooth. Place breadcrumbs in a second bowl.
5. Working one patty at a time, dip in flour mixture to coat, then transfer to breadcrumbs. Cover with breadcrumbs on all sides, and transfer to a plate. Repeat with remaining patties.
6. Put half of oil in a large cast iron or non-stick skillet over medium-high heat until shimmering. Add the patties in a single layer and cook, swirling pan occasionally, until golden brown on bottoms, about 2 minutes. Carefully flip and cook second side, swirling pan occasionally as they cook, about 2 minutes longer.
7. Place avocado in a small bowl and mash the flesh with a fork. Season with salt and add lime juice. Serve fried chickpea patties with mashed avocado, sliced onions, herbs, and lime or lemon wedges.

Nutritional Information:

Calories: 697 | Total Fat: 28 g | Carbohydrates: 96 g | Protein: 15 g

Vegan Paella

Ingredients:
130 ml boiling water
50 g white rice
¾ tsp. coconut oil
¼ onion, chopped
1 garlic clove, minced
¼ green bell pepper, sliced
¼ red bell pepper, sliced
½ tomato, diced
120 ml vegetable broth
1 tsp. paprika
½ tsp. ground turmeric
40 g peas
50 g drained and quartered canned artichoke hearts
Salt and pepper

Directions:
1. Mix boiling water and rice together in a bowl; let stand for 20 minutes. Drain.
2. Heat oil in a large skillet over medium heat; cook and stir onion and garlic until onion is transparent, about 5 minutes. Add green bell pepper, red bell pepper, and tomato; cook and stir until peppers are slightly tender, about 3 minutes.
3. Mix rice and vegetable broth into onion-pepper mixture; bring to a boil. Reduce heat to low and simmer. Add paprika, turmeric and a pinch of salt and pepper; cover skillet and simmer until rice is tender, about 20 minutes.
4. Stir peas and artichoke hearts into rice mixture and cook until heated through, about 1 minute more. Serve hot.

Nutritional Information:
Calories: 125 | Total Fat: 2 g | Carbohydrates: 26 g | Protein: 2 g

Hot Edamame-Quinoa-Mix

Ingredients:

200 ml water
65 g quinoa
1 tsp. vegetable bouillon
120 g shelled edamame
1 tsp. coconut oil
½ sweet onion, diced
½ bell pepper, diced
1 ½ tsp. minced fresh ginger
2 garlic cloves, minced
1 Tbsp. soy sauce
2 tsp. chopped fresh cilantro
1 tsp. Sriracha, or other hot chili paste

Directions:

1. Bring water, quinoa, and vegetable bouillon to a boil in a medium pot; stir in edamame, cover, and simmer until quinoa is tender, 15 to 20 minutes.
2. Heat oil in a medium skillet over medium heat; cook and stir onions and bell peppers until onions are translucent, about 5 minutes.
3. Add ginger and garlic; cook and stir until fragrant, about 2 minutes. Remove from heat; stir in soy sauce, cilantro, and chili paste.
4. Combine onion mixture and quinoa mixture; simmer, stirring occasionally, until excess broth has been absorbed, about 5 minutes. Serve.

Nutritional Information:

Calories: 166 | Total Fat: 5 g | Carbohydrates: 21 g | Protein: 9 g

Avocado Pasta Mix

Ingredients:
Veggies:
¼ head broccoli, cut into 1-inch/2 cm florets
½ red bell pepper, cut into ½ inch/1 cm chunks
¼ yellow onion, thinly sliced into rings
2 tsp. coconut oil
Juice from half a lime
Pinch of salt
Sauce:
1 avocado, peeled and chopped
Juice from ½ lime
1 garlic clove, peeled
2 Tbsp. chopped fresh cilantro
Salt and pepper
Pasta:
150 g penne pasta
Pinch of salt

Directions:
1. Preheat oven to 450°F/230°C. Combine broccoli, red bell peppers, and yellow onion in a large bowl. Add oil, juice from ½ a lime, and a pinch of salt; toss to coat. Spread vegetables onto a baking sheet.
2. Roast vegetables for 30 minutes, stirring 1 or 2 times, until edges begin to blacken. Remove from oven and cool slightly.
3. Fill a large pot with water and a pinch of salt; bring to a boil. Stir in penne and return to a boil. Cook pasta uncovered, stirring occasionally, until cooked through but still firm to the bite, about 11 minutes; drain.
4. Blend avocado, juice from ½ a lime, garlic, and pinch of salt and pepper in a food processor or blender until sauce is smooth, scraping down sides as needed. Add chopped cilantro and pulse until just incorporated.
5. Gently toss pasta, roasted vegetables, and sauce together in a bowl. Serve.

Nutritional Information:
Calories: 327 | Total Fat: 12 g | Carbohydrates: 46 g | Protein: 10 g

Quinoa Pilaf

Ingredients:
1 tsp. extra virgin coconut oil
1 Tbsp. onion, diced
1 clove garlic, minced
40 g uncooked quinoa, rinsed
2 Tbsp. canned/prepared lentils, rinsed
130 ml vegetable broth
¼ bunch Swiss chard, stems removed

Directions:
1. Heat the oil in a small pot over medium heat. Stir in the onion and garlic, and sauté until onion is tender, about 5 minutes.
2. Add in quinoa and lentils. Pour in the broth. Cover, and cook 15 minutes.
3. Remove the pot from heat. Shred chard, and gently mix into the pot. Cover, and allow to sit 5 minutes, or until chard is wilted.
4. Serve and enjoy.

Nutritional Information:
Calories: 149 | Total Fat: 3 g | Carbohydrates: 27 g | Protein: 4 g

Broccoli Quiche

Ingredients:
1 (9-inch/23 cm) unbaked vegan pie crust
1 large head of broccoli, chopped
1 Tbsp. coconut oil
1 onion, finely chopped
4 cloves garlic, minced
500 g firm tofu, drained
130 ml soy milk (or preferred milk alternative)
¼ tsp. Dijon mustard
¾ tsp. salt
¼ tsp. ground nutmeg
½ tsp. ground red pepper
Black pepper to taste
1 Tbsp. dried parsley
20 g parmesan flavour soy cheese

Directions:
1. Preheat oven to 400°F/200°C. Bake pie crust in preheated oven for 10 to 12 minutes.
2. Place broccoli in a steamer over 1 inch/2 cm of boiling water and cover. Cook until tender but still firm, about 2 to 6 minutes. Drain and set aside.
3. Heat oil in a large skillet over medium-high heat. Sauté onion and garlic until golden, about 3-5 minutes. Stir in the broccoli and cook for an additional minute.
4. In a blender, combine tofu, soy milk, mustard, salt, nutmeg, ground red pepper, black pepper, parsley and Parmesan soy cheese and blend until smooth.
5. In a large bowl combine tofu mixture with broccoli mixture. Pour into pie crust.
6. Bake in preheated oven until quiche is set, about 35 to 40 minutes. Allow to stand for at least 5 minutes before cutting and serving. Leftovers can be stored in an airtight container in the fridge for up to a week.

Nutritional Information (for 1/6th of quiche):
Calories: 354 | Total Fat: 20 g | Carbohydrates: 26 g | Protein: 18 g

Baked Lentils with Rice

Ingredients:
100 g long-grain rice, uncooked
650 ml water
200 g red lentils
1 tsp. coconut oil
1 small onion, diced
3 cloves garlic, minced
1 tomato, diced
35 g diced celery
40 g chopped carrots
50 g chopped zucchini
240 g tomato sauce
1 tsp. dried basil
1 tsp. dried oregano
1 tsp. ground cumin
½ tsp. celery seed
Salt and pepper, to taste

Directions:
1. Preheat oven to 350°F/180°C. In a small bowl, combine basil, oregano, cumin, celery seed, and a pinch of salt and pepper. Set aside.
2. Place the rice and 300 ml of water in a medium pot over high heat and bring to a boil. Cover, reduce heat to low, and simmer 20 minutes.
3. Place lentils in a pot with the remaining water, and bring to a boil. Cook 15 minutes, or until tender. Heat the oil in a skillet over medium heat, and stir in the onion and garlic. Mix in tomato, celery, carrots, zucchini, and ½ the tomato sauce. Season with ½ the seasoning mix.
4. In a casserole dish, mix the rice, lentils, and vegetables. Top with remaining tomato sauce, and sprinkle with remaining seasoning.
5. Bake 30 minutes in the preheated oven, until the top is bubbling. Remove and serve. Store leftovers in an airtight container, in the fridge, for up to a week.

Nutritional Information (for 1/6th of bake):
Calories: 193 | Total Fat: 2 g | Carbohydrates: 35 g | Protein: 10 g

Black Bean Quesadillas

Ingredients:

100 g great Northern beans, drained and rinsed

4 Tbsp. diced tomatoes

1 clove garlic, minced

½ tsp. ground cumin

Pinch of chili powder

Pinch cayenne pepper

40 g black beans, drained and rinsed

Pinch of salt

2 whole grain tortillas

1 Tbsp. fresh, chopped cilantro

1 tsp. coconut oil

Directions:

1. Blend great Northern beans, 3 Tbsp. tomatoes, and garlic in a food processor until smooth; add cumin, chili powder, pinch of salt and cayenne and blend again.
2. Transfer bean mixture to a bowl. Stir black beans, 1 Tbsp. tomatoes, and cilantro into bean mixture.
3. Heat oil in skillet over medium-high heat. Place a tortilla in the hot oil. Spread about bean filling onto the tortilla.
4. Place another tortilla on top of filling; cook until filling is warmed, about 10 minutes.
5. Flip quesadilla to cook the second side until lightly browned, 3 to 5 minutes.

Nutritional Information:

Calories: 122 | Total Fat: 2 g | Carbohydrates: 21 g | Protein: 6 g

Stuffed Bell Pepper

Ingredients:
50 g brown rice
120 ml water
1 red bell pepper, top and seeds removed
1 tsp coconut oil
¼ onion, chopped
1 garlic clove, chopped
100 g can black-eyed peas, rinsed and drained
1 large Swiss Chard leaf, chopped
Salt and pepper, to taste

Directions:
1. Preheat oven to 350°F/180°C. Spray a baking sheet with cooking spray or grease with cooking oil.
2. Bring the brown rice and water to a boil in a saucepan over high heat. Reduce the heat to medium-low, cover, and simmer until the rice is tender and the liquid has been absorbed, 15-30 minutes.
3. Place the red pepper on the prepared baking sheet, and bake until tender, about 15 minutes.
4. Heat the oil in a skillet over medium heat, cook and stir the onion and garlic until the onion is translucent, about 5 minutes.
5. Stir in the black-eyed peas and chard. Bring the mixture to a simmer, and cook until the chard is wilted, 5 to 8 minutes. Mix in the cooked brown rice, sprinkle with salt and pepper to taste, and lightly stuff the mixture into the red pepper. Serve hot.

Nutritional Information:
Calories: 100 | Total Fat: 1 g | Carbohydrates: 21 g | Protein: 2 g

Couscous with Olives and Tomatoes

Ingredients:
120 ml vegetable broth, divided
60 ml water
90 g pearl couscous
Pinch salt and pepper
1 Tbsp. coconut oil
2 Tbsp. pine nuts
1 clove garlic, minced
¼ shallot, minced
2 Tbsp. sliced black olives
1 Tbsp. sun- dried tomatoes packed in oil, drained and chopped
1 Tbsp. chopped fresh parsley

Directions:
1. Bring 60 ml vegetable broth and water to a boil in a saucepan, stir in couscous, and mix in salt and black pepper. Reduce heat to low and simmer until liquid is absorbed, about 8 minutes.
2. Heat 1 tsp. oil in a skillet over medium-high heat; stir in pine nuts and cook, stirring frequently, until pine nuts smell toasted and are golden brown, about 1 minute. Remove from heat.
3. Heat remaining 1 Tbsp. oil in a saucepan; cook and stir garlic and shallot in the hot oil until softened, about 2 minutes. Stir black olives and sun-dried tomatoes into garlic mixture and cook until heated through, 2 to 3 minutes, stirring often.
4. Slowly pour in remaining vegetable broth and bring mixture to a boil. Reduce heat to low and simmer until sauce has reduced, 8 to 10 minutes.
5. Transfer couscous to a bowl, mix with sauce, and serve topped with parsley and pine nuts.

Nutritional Information:
Calories: 142 | Total Fat: 7 g | Carbohydrates: 16 g | Protein: 3 g

Carrot Soup Curry Style

Ingredients:
1 tsp. coconut oil
1 tsp. curry powder
1 garlic clove, smashed
¼ inch/0.5 cm piece of ginger, peeled and smashed
¼ medium onion, coarsely chopped
2 carrots, peeled and sliced into ¼ inch/0.5 cm thick rounds
1 bay leaf
250 ml vegetable broth
60 ml coconut milk

Directions:
1. Heat the oil in a medium saucepan over medium heat. When it shimmers, add the curry powder and garlic and cook until fragrant, about 30 seconds.
2. Add the ginger, onion, carrots, bay leaf, and broth, increase the heat to medium high, and bring the mixture to a boil. Reduce the heat to medium low and simmer until the carrots are soft when pierced with a fork, about 20 minutes. Discard the bay leaf.
3. Working in batches, process the soup in a blender until smooth. (Be careful when blending the hot soup, as steam could blow off the blender lid.)
4. Pour the soup into a clean pot and return it to the stove over medium heat. Stir in the coconut milk and adjust the seasoning as needed. Serve hot.

Nutritional Information:
Calories: 250 | Total Fat: 13 g | Carbohydrates: 30 g | Protein: 3 g

Image sources/Printing information
Pictures cover: depositphotos.com;
@ marcomayer; @ Paul_Cowan; @ Esbenklinker; @ daffodil
This print edition:
IngramSpark – Lightning Source LLC
ISBN (paperback glossy): 978-3-98500-309-9
BuchHörnchen-Verlag
Im Schlimm 13
55768 Hoppstädten-Weiersbach (Germany)